UNDO CHRONIC KIDNEY DISEASE

The Plant Based Remedy

By

Dr. Stacy Rose

Remarks

This is a good book for anyone battling with kidney disease, it's more of a splendid guide.

Rita Stacy, PhD

I like the way Stacy writes her stuff like it's a lecture note.

Sandra cook, CEO, BLU

Short, precise and straight to the point.

Natalie Freeman, Actress

CONTENTS

INTRODUCTION

UNDERSTANDING KIDNEY DISEASE

Chronic kidney disease, as it was generally named — is a term that incorporates all levels of diminished kidney capability, from harmed kidneys to serious ongoing kidney failure. Chronict kidney illness is an overall general medical condition. In the US, there is a rising rate and commonness of kidney failure.

Chronic kidney disease is more common in the aged population. Close to half of the patients with chronic kidney disease are more than 70 years of age. Nonetheless, while more youthful patients with chronic kidney disease commonly experience moderate loss of kidney capability, 30% of patients near 65 years old have this illness.

Every year, only a couple of youngsters out of each 100,000 - who are 19 years of age or more youthful -

experience kidney failure. By examination, adults are multiple times bound to foster kidney failure than youngsters, with the risk expanding consistently with age.

Besides, African Americans in their late adolescents are multiple times more probable than Caucasians in a similar age to have kidney failure, as well as illnesses that harm the little veins in the kidney. What's more, young men are almost two times as likely as young ladies to have kidney failure from birth complications, polycystic kidney sickness, or other genetic infections. The Dialysis Center at Cincinnati Children's Hospital gives data to patients and families to more readily comprehend kidney capability, kidney failure - both acute and persistent.

CKD is a condition wherein the kidneys are harmed and can't channel blood along with them. Along these lines, an abundance of liquid and waste from blood stay in the body and may cause other medical conditions, like coronary illness and stroke.

CKD has degrees of seriousness. It typically looks more terrible after some time however treatment has been displayed to slow its diminishing effect. Whenever left untreated, CKD can advance to kidney failure and early cardiovascular infection. At the point when the kidneys quit working, dialysis or kidney relocation is required for endurance. Kidney failure treated with dialysis or surgery is called end-stage renal illness.

Not all patients with kidney illness progress to kidney failure. To assist with forestalling CKD and bring down the risk for kidney failure, control risk factors for CKD, get experimented yearly, perform way of life changes, take medication depending on the situation, and see your medical services group routinely.

It's a condition frequently connected with aging. It can affect anybody, however it's more considered normal in individuals who are dark or of south Asian origin. CKD can deteriorate after some time and in the end the kidneys might quit working, yet this is not common. Many people with CKD can carry on with long lives with the condition.

CHAPTER ONE

THE RELEVANCE OF KIDNEY HEALTH

In ancient period of history, the kidneys were seen as the seat of emotion, feeling and desires and the wellspring of profound morality and good action. The kidneys were connected with the deepest pieces of an individual's character. While we know since kidneys play no immediate part in molding our morals, feelings and character, these two bean-formed organs are regardless essential to our health.

The kidney is a strikingly multifaceted organ that goes about as the channeling aspect of the body. Similarly as significant, your kidneys likewise work to keep the entire body in a condition of substance balance. The kidneys manage the substances, helpful and toxic that float around in the body and keep them inside extremely

close boundaries so the body can work as a perfectly orchestrated system. This is called renal workings.
You can't survive without good renal working regardless of whether the kidneys are aided artificially. Life wouldn't go on without the many capabilities these organs perform.
The kidney is the central part in the guideline of your pulse, and the make-up of the blood. Keeping up with a huge number that are indispensable to our actual presence, the kidneys even produce chemicals that let bones know when to make more platelets.

People are a complicated and coordinated creation and the kidneys work with your other organs to assist you with carrying on with a sound life. Tragically, when one organ or framework fails to work appropriately, others can start to diminish subsequently.
when the kidneys waver, numerous life changing issues can result.
Like any complex machine, the kidney is profoundly delicate to its current circumstance. Each time our heart beats, the kidneys get around 20% of the blood that is siphoned. In the event that the kidneys don't get sufficient blood, they will begin to disintegrate. Numerous intense ailments, which are illnesses or ailments with extreme or unexpected beginning, can cause blood flow to fall. So it's exceptionally considered

normal to have intense kidney injury at whatever point we get intensely sick.

Your kidneys are one of the important organ in your body. Thus, their wellbeing ought to be really important as you make way of life changes and foster healthy behavior. We should investigate the significance of our kidneys and how you can guarantee yours are healthy.

Great kidney wellbeing is significant in light of the fact that it helps keep your whole body working appropriately. Probably the most widely recognized issues related with unfortunate kidney wellbeing include:

- Hypertension.
- Chronic kidney disease
- Kidney diseases brought about by microorganisms or infections.
- Loss of kidney capability because of parchedness, diabetes, urinary plot diseases, and other ailments.

Perceiving issues with your kidney almost immediately can assist with the early recognition of additional difficult circumstances like kidney infection. In the event that you experience any of the accompanying side effects, it is essential to get looked at by a specialist immediately:

- Dull urine
- Expanding in lower legs or feet.
- Pain toward the back or side of the kidneys.
- Great exhaustion.
- Trouble peeing or continuous pee

It's essential to deal with your kidneys by ensuring you stay hydrated, eat a solid, adjusted diet, and endeavor to routinely work-out. Furthermore, it's really smart to remove propensities like smoking and inordinate liquor utilization, as these can overwork and damage your kidneys in the long run.

At long last, deal with your kidneys by going to your consistently planned specialist's visits. These visits are intended to assist with keeping up with your general wellbeing and recognize any issues as soon as conceivable to start treatment and get a course for better wellbeing.

Your kidneys are clenched and estimated organs situated at the lower part of your rib, on the two sides of your spine. They carry out a few roles.

In particular, they channel side-effects, overabundance of water, and different contaminations from your blood. These byproducts are put away in your bladder and later removed through pee.

What's more, your kidneys manage pH, salt, and potassium levels in your body. They additionally produce chemicals that manage circulatory strain and control the creation of red platelets.

Your kidneys are likewise answerable for enacting a type of vitamin D that assists your body with engrossing calcium for building bones and managing muscle capability.

Keeping up with kidney health means a lot to your general wellbeing. By keeping your kidneys healthy, your body will channel appropriately and produce chemicals to assist your body with working appropriately.

Here are a few hints to assist with keeping your kidneys solid.

1. Be active and fit

Regular activity is not just for your waistline. It can bring down the risk of constant kidney illness. It can likewise diminish your pulse and lift your heart health, which are both significant for forestalling kidney harm. You don't need to partake in long distance races to receive the benefit of exercising. Strolling, running, cycling, and in any event, moving are perfect for your wellbeing. Find a movement that keeps you occupied and have some good times. It'll be simpler to keep up with it and have extraordinary outcomes.

2. Deal with your glucose

Individuals with diabetes, or a condition that causes high glucose, may foster kidney harm. At the point when your body's cells can't break down the glucose (sugar) in your blood, your kidneys are compelled to endeavor to direct your blood. Over long periods of effort, this can prompt dangerous harm.
Be that as it may, on the off chance that you can deal with your glucose, you lessen the risk of harm. Likewise, in the event that the harm is gotten early, a specialist can do whatever it takes to diminish or forestall extra harm.

3. Study your blood pressure

Hypertension can cause kidney harm. Assuming hypertension happens with other medical problems like diabetes, coronary illness, or elevated cholesterol, the effect on your body can be huge.
A healthy circulatory strain perusing is 120/80. Prehypertension is between that point and 139/89. Way of life and dietary changes might assist with bringing down your pulse as of now.

Assuming your circulatory strain readings are reliably over 140/90, you might have hypertension. You ought to consult with a specialist about observing your circulatory strain consistently, making changes to your way of life, and perhaps taking medicine.

4. Study your weight and eat a balanced diet

Individuals who are obese or have heftiness are in danger of various medical issues that can harm the kidneys. These incorporate diabetes, coronary illness, and kidney disease.
A reasonable eating plan that is low in sodium, processed meats, and other kidney-harming food sources might assist with decreasing the risk of kidney harm. Center around eating new fixings that are normally low in sodium, like cauliflower, blueberries, fish, entire grains, from there, the sky's the limit.

5. Drink a lot of liquids

It is advisable to drink at least 8 glasses of water per day.
yet it's a decent objective unequivocally on the grounds
that it urges you to remain hydrated. Ordinary, steady
water intake is good for your kidneys.
Water helps remove sodium and poisons from your
kidneys. It likewise brings down your risk of ongoing
kidney sickness.
At Least 1.5 to 2 liters in a day. Precisely how much
water you want relies to a great extent upon your health
and way of life. Factors like environment, work out,
orientation, in general wellbeing, and whether you're
pregnant or breastfeeding are critical to consider while
arranging your everyday water consumption.
Individuals who have recently had kidney stones ought
to hydrate to assist with forestalling stone stores from
here on out.

6. Try not to smoke

Smoking harms your body's veins. This prompts a
slower blood stream all through your body and to your
kidneys.
Smoking additionally puts your kidneys at an expanded
gamble for disease. Assuming you smoke and quit

smoking, your risk will drop. Nonetheless, it'll require numerous years to get back to the risk level of a smoker.

CHAPTER TWO:

CAUSES OF CHRONIC KIDNEY DISEASE

Diabetes and hypertension are the most widely recognized reasons for constant kidney disease (CKD). Your medical specialist will take a look at your health history and may do tests to figure out why you have kidney illness. The reason for your kidney disease might influence the sort of treatment you get.

Diabetes

A lot of glucose, likewise called sugar, in your blood harms your kidneys' channels. Over the long run, your kidneys can turn out to be harmed to the point that they never again work really hard separating wastes and additional liquid from your blood. Frequently, the principal indication of kidney disease from diabetes is protein in your pee. At the point when the channels are harmed, a protein called egg whites, which you want to remain solid, drops off your blood and into your pee. A solid kidney doesn't allow egg whites to pass from the blood into the pee. Diabetic kidney sickness is the clinical term for kidney illness brought about by diabetes.

Hypertension

Hypertension can harm veins in the kidneys so they don't fill in also. In the event that the veins in your kidneys are harmed, your kidneys may not function too well to eliminate wastes and additional liquid from your body.

Additional liquid in the veins may then raise circulatory strain considerably more, making a hazardous cycle.

Glomerulonephritis: Glomerulonephritis is a gathering of illnesses that cause irritation and harm the kidney's separating units. These problems are the third most normal sort of kidney sickness.

Heredity: Polycystic kidney sickness, or PKD, is a typical acquired illness that makes huge pimples structure in the kidneys and harm the encompassing tissue.

Kidney and urinary parcel anomalies before birth

Mutations that happen as a child creates in its mom's belly. For instance, a limitation might happen that forestalls ordinary surge of pee and makes pee stream back up to the kidney. This causes contaminations and may harm the kidneys.
Immune system illnesses: At the point when the body's guard framework, the resistant framework, betrays the body, it's called an immune system illness. Lupus nephritis is one such immune system sickness that results

in irritation (enlarging or scarring) of the little veins that channel squanders in your kidney.

Impediments brought about by kidney stones or growths can cause kidney harm. An augmented prostate organ in men or rehashed urinary diseases can likewise cause kidney harm.

What are the side effects?

A great many people might not have any extreme side effects until their kidney illness has progressed. In any scenario, you might notice that you:

- feel more drained and have less energy
- experience difficulty concentrating
- have a decreased appetite
- experience difficulty dozing
- have muscle cramps around evening time
- have enlarged feet and ankles
- have puffiness around your eyes, particularly toward the beginning of the day
- have dry, irritated skin
- need to pee on a more regular basis, particularly around evening time.

CHAPTER THREE: LEVELS OF CHRONIC KIDNEY DISEASE

Kidneys have many positions crucial to great wellbeing. They go about as channels for your blood, eliminating waste, poisons, and surplus liquids.

There are five phases of CKD, and various side effects and medicines are related to each stage.

Stage 1 kidney disease

In stage 1, there's extremely gentle harm to the kidneys. They're very versatile and can adapt to this, permitting them to continue to perform at 90% or better.

At this stage, CKD is probably going to be found by chance during routine blood and pee tests. You may likewise have these tests assuming that you have diabetes or hypertension, the top reasons for CKD in the US.

Side effects

Commonly, there are no side effects when kidneys are at 90% or better.

Treatment

You can slow infection movement by making these strides:

- Work at overseeing glucose levels on the off chance that you have diabetes.
- Heed your primary care physician's guidance for bringing down circulatory strain assuming that you have hypertension.
- Keep a solid, adjusted diet.
- Try not to utilize tobacco.
- Take part in actual work for 30 minutes per day, no less than 5 days per week.
- Attempt to keep a proper weight

Stage 2 kidney disease

In stage 2 CKD, kidneys are working between 60 - 89%.

Side effects

At this stage, you could in any case be side effect free.
Or on the other hand side effects are vague, for example,
- exhaustion
- tingling
- loss of craving
- rest problems
- Weakness

Treatment

There's no solution for CKD, however early treatment
can slow or stop movement
Tending to the hidden cause is fundamental. In the event
that you have diabetes, hypertension, or coronary illness,
adhere to your PCP's guidelines for dealing with these
circumstances.
It's likewise critical to keep a decent eating regimen,
work-out routinely, and oversee weight. Assuming you
smoke, get some information about smoking suspension
programs.

Stage 3 kidney disease

Stage 3A CKD implies your kidney is working between 45 - 59%. Stage 3B means kidney capability is between 30 - 44%
The kidneys aren't separating waste, poisons, and liquids well, which are beginning to develop.

Side effects

Not every person has side effects at stage 3. In any case, you might have:
- Pain at the back
- weariness
- loss of hunger
- Persistent tingling
- rest issues
- expanding of the hands and feet
- peeing pretty much than expected
- Weakness

Complications

- Anemia
- hypertension
- Hypertension

Treatment

It's critical to oversee basic circumstances to assist with saving kidney capability. This might include:

- hypertension meds, for example, angiotensin-changing over compound (Expert) inhibitors or angiotensin II receptor blockers
- diuretics and a low-salt eating routine to ease liquid maintenance
- cholesterol-reducing drugs
- erythropoietin drugs for anemia
- vitamin D enhancements to address debilitating bones
- phosphate folios to forestall calcification in the veins
- following a lower protein diet so your kidneys don't need to fill in as hard

You'll presumably require continuous subsequent visits and tests, so changes can be made if vital.

Stage 4 kidney disease

Stage 4 CKD implies you have moderate-to-serious kidney harm. They're working between 15 - 29%, so you might develop more waste, poisons, and liquids in your body.

You should give your best for forestall movement to kidney disappointment.

As per the Habitats for Infectious prevention and Prevention(CDC), 40% of individuals with seriously diminished kidney capability aren't even mindful they have it.

Side effects

Side effects can include:
- back pain
- chest pain
- diminished mental sharpness
- weariness
- loss of hunger
- muscle jerks or spasms
- queasiness and spewing
- relentless tingling
- windedness
- rest issues
- enlarging of the hands and feet
- peeing pretty much than expected

Intricacies can include:

- frailty

- bone illness
- hypertension
-

You're likewise at an expanded chance of coronary illness and stroke.

Treatment

In stage 4, you should work intimately with your PCPs. Notwithstanding similar treatment as prior stages, you ought to begin conversations about dialysis and kidney relocate should your kidneys come up short.
These strategies take cautious association and a ton of time, so beginning anticipating them with your primary care physician however ahead of schedule as possible seems to be insightful.
Moreover, stage 4 CKD can prompt further unexpected problems requiring treatment. For instance, it is entirely expected for individuals to foster metabolic acidosis because of CKD. Contingent upon blood bicarbonate levels, specialists might recommend oral bicarbonate substitution treatment.

Stage 5 kidney disease

Stage 5 CKD implies your kidneys are working at under 15% limit, or you have kidney disappointment.

At the point when that occurs, the development of waste and poisons becomes hazardous. This is end-stage renal sickness.

Side effects

Side effects of kidney failure can include:

- back and chest pain
- breathing issues
- diminished mental sharpness
- exhaustion
- practically zero craving
- muscle jerks or issues
- queasiness or spewing
- tingling
- inconvenience resting
- serious weakness
- enlarging of the hands and feet
- peeing pretty much than expected

CHAPTER FOUR

DIETS AND NUTRITION GUIDE FOR KIDNEY HEALTH

A kidney-accommodating eating plan ought to restrict sodium, cholesterol, and fat, and on second thought center around organic products, vegetables, whole grains, low-fat dairy, and lean meats (fish, poultry, eggs, vegetables, nuts, seeds, and soy items), says Maruschak. Individuals who have previously been determined to have CKD may likewise have to restrict specific different supplements, she adds.

The following are a couple of ways of redesigning your eating routine to keep up with kidney wellbeing.

Limit Your Salt Consumption

Sodium slips its direction into a wide range of direction you wouldn't envision, particularly packaged food varieties like soups and breads. Restricting your sodium consumption helps keep your blood under control — that is around 1 teaspoon of table salt — as per the Dietary Rules for Americans, 2020-2025, distributed by the U.S. Division of Agribusiness (USDA).

Be Aware of Protein

At the point when you eat protein, your body produces waste that is separated through your kidneys. While protein is a significant piece of a solid eating plan, eating more protein than you want might make your kidneys work harder. While research on the impacts of a high-protein diet on generally speaking kidney wellbeing is as yet developing, as verified in a review from 2020, your primary care physician will probably suggest a lower-protein diet in the event that you as of now have CKD. " Having a lot of protein can make waste develop in your blood, and your kidneys will be unable to eliminate it," Maruschak says.

Individuals with any phase of CKD who aren't on dialysis ought to restrict their protein consumption to 0.6 to 0.8 grams per kilogram of body weight to diminish kidney infection movement, Maruschak says. For instance, an individual who weighs 150 pounds (68kg) would require 40 to 54 grams of protein each day, which is around 4 to 6 ounces of protein from creature or plant sources, as indicated by the Public Kidney Groundwork of Hawaii. Make certain to talk with an enrolled dietitian to decide the perfect proportion of protein for you.

Limit Saturated fats and Stay away from Trans Fat

Eat less trans fats because it increases the risk of coronary illness — and what's terrible for your heart is awful for your kidneys. " Heart wellbeing and kidney wellbeing are interconnected, as the heart continually siphons blood all through the body and the kidneys ceaselessly channel the blood to eliminate side-effects and an abundance of liquid from the body," Maruschak says.

The USDA's dietary rules prescribe restricting saturated fats to under 10% of your complete everyday calories. Fundamental sources incorporate meats, full-fat dairy items, butter, fat, coconut oil, and palm oil, says Maruschak. What's more, attempt to keep away from trans fats, tracked down in prepared merchandise and seared food sources. All things being equal, top off on heart-solid unsaturated fats, tracked down in fatty fish, avocados, olives, walnuts, and many kinds of vegetable oils.

Watch Your Alcohol intake

Alcohol hurts your kidneys in more ways than one, which makes sense to Maruschak. It's a side-effect that your kidneys need to sift through your blood — and it makes your kidneys less productive. It's drying out, which can influence the kidneys' capacity to manage your body's water levels. It can influence your liver capability, which thus can affect blood flow to the kidneys and lead to CKD after some time. Furthermore, a high liquor consumption has been connected to an expanded risk of hypertension, which can prompt kidney illness.

Maruschak says all kinds of people ought to drink something like one cocktail each day. That is 12 ounces of normal brew, 5 ounces of wine, or 1.5 ounces (a single shot glass) of refined spirits, as per the Public Establishment on Liquor Misuse and Liquor abuse. " It's best to talk with your doctor about your liquor consumption, as certain individuals ought not to be taking off any liquor whatsoever," she says.

Quality Nourishment For Individuals With KIDNEY Disease

. Red peppers

Half cup serving red bell pepper = 1 milligram sodium, 88 milligram potassium, 10 milligram phosphorus

Red bell peppers are low in potassium and much in flavor, yet that is not by any means the only explanation they're ideally suited for the kidney diet. These delicious vegetables are likewise a fantastic sources of nutrients C and A, as well as vitamin B6, folic corrosive and fiber. Red ringer peppers are great for you since they contain lycopene, a cell reinforcement that helps safeguards against specific tumors.

You can likewise cook peppers and use them as a garnish on sandwiches or lettuce plates of mixed greens, hack them for an omelet, add them to kabobs on the barbecue or stuff peppers with ground turkey or meat and prepare them for a principal dish.

Cabbage

Half cup serving green cabbage = 6 milligram sodium, 60 mg potassium, 9 milligram phosphorus

A cruciferous vegetable, cabbage is pressed brimming with phytochemicals, the substance intensifies in natural products or vegetables that separates free extremists before they can cause harm. Numerous phytochemicals are likewise known to assist with shielding cells from harm that could prompt malignant growth, as well as cultivate cardiovascular wellbeing.

High in vitamin K, L-ascorbic acid and fiber, cabbage is likewise a decent wellspring of vitamin B6 and folic corrosive. Lower in potassium and lower in cost, it's a reasonable expansion to the kidney diet.

Crude cabbage makes an extraordinary expansion to the dialysis diet as coleslaw or a garnish for fish tacos. You can steam, microwave or bubble it, add spread or cream cheddar in addition to pepper or caraway seeds and serve it as a side dish. Cabbage Rolls Made with Turkey are an extraordinary tidbit, and on the off chance that you're feeling extravagant, you can stuff a cabbage with ground meat and prepare it for a tasty dinner overflowing with supplements.

Garlic

Garlic has antimicrobial properties that assist with keeping plaque from shaping on your teeth, brings down cholesterol and diminishes irritation.

Get it new, packaged, minced or powdered, and add it to meat, vegetable or pasta dishes. You can likewise cook a head of garlic and spread it on bread. Garlic gives a tasty flavor and garlic powder is an extraordinary substitute for garlic salt in the dialysis diet.

Apples

1 medium apple with skin = 0 sodium, 158 milligram potassium, 10 milligram phosphorus

Apples might assist with lessening cholesterol, forestall clogging, safeguard against coronary illness and diminish the gamble of disease. High in fiber and calming compounds, an apple daily may truly assist with fending the specialist off — uplifting news for individuals with kidney illness who as of now have their portion of specialist visits.

This kidney diet fruit can be matched with the previous really great for-you food, onions, to make an exceptional Apple Onion Omelet. Apples are flexible. You can eat them raw, make heated apples, stew apples, make them into fruit purée, or drink them as squeezed apple or apple juice.

Red grapes

Red grapes contain a few flavonoids that give them a red color. Flavonoids help safeguard against heart disease by forestalling oxidation and lessening the arrangement of blood clusters. Resveratrol, a flavonoid tracked down in grapes, may likewise animate creation of nitric oxide which loosens up muscle cells in the veins to increment blood stream. These flavonoids likewise give insurance against disease and assist with forestalling aggravation.

Purchase grapes with red or purple skin since their anthocyanin content is higher. Freeze them to eat as a bite or to extinguish hunger for those on a liquid limitation for the dialysis diet. Add grapes to a natural product salad or chicken plate of mixed greens. Try an extraordinary kidney diet recipe for Turkey Kabobs that highlights grapes. You can likewise drink them as grape juice.

Egg whites

Egg whites are unadulterated protein and give great protein to every one of the fundamental amino acids. For the kidney diet, egg whites give protein less phosphorus than other protein sources like egg yolk or meats.

Purchase powdered, new or pasteurized egg whites. Make an omelet or egg white sandwich, add purified egg whites to smoothies or shakes, make spiced egg snacks, or add whites of hard-bubbled eggs to fish salad or nursery salad to add additional protein.

Olive oil

Olive oil is an extraordinary wellspring of oleic acid, a calming unsaturated fat. The monounsaturated fat in olive oil safeguards against oxidation. Olive oil is rich in polyphenols and cell reinforcement intensifies forestall aggravation and oxidation.

 Studies show that populations that utilize a lot of olive oil rather than different oils have lower rates of heart disease.

Exercise and kidney disease

Physical activity is critical to keeping up with your general wellbeing. This doesn't mean running a long distance race - there are numerous things that count towards active work like strolling, cycling, planting or other coincidental activity, like shopping or playing with your children or grandchildren.

Showing improvement over doing none, so in the event that you're uncertain about what you can accomplish, begin with modest quantities and gradually develop after some time.

Being physical might turn out to be more troublesome as your sickness advances, yet it's still vital. Attempt to consider active work your routine at every possible opportunity and consider it part of your treatment.

CHAPTER FIVE: PLANT BASED REMEDY FOR CHRONIC KIDNEY DISEASE

Another review published on November, 4, 2022, has approved more nearby plants for the anticipation and treatment of kidney diseases. Top on the rundown is ginger, grape, turmeric, beetroot juice, stinging bramble, onions, apples, tea, papaya, severe leaf, and guava leaves.

Plants, green growth and organisms have been used as normal meds all through mankind's set of experiences. Restorative plants are viewed as a satisfactory, modest, effectively accessible and somewhat safe wellspring of numerous dynamic mixtures for drugs. In China, the utilization of customary home grown medication for kidney illness enjoys a few upper hands over single traditional medication treatment. The helpful impact of restorative plants on kidney diseases is frequently gotten from their capacity to support the normal cancer prevention agent guard systems in the body. Various sorts of phytochemicals like flavonoids, nutrients, resveratrol, anthocyanin, curcumin and phenolic corrosive are much of the time found in plant-based meds and may go about as cancer prevention agents.

Ginger is utilized generally as a spice yet additionally frequently in society medication. It has a place with the Zingiberaceae family and has been developed for millennia, particularly in China and South Asian nations. Ginger contains numerous helpful mixtures, the most significant of which are 6-, 8-, and 10-gingerol and 6-shogaol. It shows assorted useful organic activities because of its strong cell reinforcement, calming, hostile to growth, against diabetic and neuroprotective exercises.

In preclinical animal type of kidney and cardiovascular illnesses, ginger concentrates brought down blood glucose levels, reestablished the absolute starches, pyruvate, glycogen and complete protein in kidney tissue, advanced the recovery of tubules and reestablished glomeruli, and diminished greasy penetration. One clinical preliminary of ginger concentrate in CKD patients on peritoneal dialysis showed that everyday organization of 1000 mg ginger diminished serum fasting glucose, a gamble factor for diabetes, diabetic nephropathy and cardiovascular sickness. There have been no unfriendly secondary effects detailed when dosages are kept to a moderate level.

For instance, rutin may prompt protein-energy unhealthiness in CKD. In spite of the fact that there are a few promising outcomes, more breaks down are expected to affirm whether, or not, preclinical and clinical advantages exist for this plant separately, especially with regards to CKD.

Clinically, Glycyrrhiza glabra separates reliably diminished pre-dialysis serum potassium fixations in ongoing hemodialysis patients. Silybum marianum, known as "milk thorn" or silymarin, is an exceptionally protected spice that safeguards against kidney disappointment and end-stage diabetic nephropathy. Huge advantages have been asserted for Lespedeza color for both AKI and CKD patients.

Clinically, beetroot juice diminished fringe systolic and diastolic circulatory strain, mean blood vessel pressure, further developed kidney capability, histological harm and kidney forecast, and forestalled cardiovascular occasions.

Rhubarb, from the base of Rheum spp native to Asia, has a place with the Polygonaceae family. A few animal categories are developed for their capability to treat CKD. Rhubarb contains mixtures like saponins, flavonoids, unstable oils, polysaccharides, tannins, stilbene glycosides (resveratrol and piceatannol) and anthraquinone glycosides (physcion, aloe-emodin, chrysophanol, emodin and rhein). The anthraquinone glycosides might have a few inborn poison levels, yet they can be eliminated from concentrates to create a successful concentrate that is nephroprotective. Numerous clinical and pre-clinical preliminaries have reliably demonstrated the way that concentrates of rhubarb can lessen serum creatinine levels and offset other metabolic brokenness connected with kidney disappointment.

In CKD treatment, rhubarb expands the discharge of nitrogenous and other byproducts through the digestive system and enhances uremic poison collection, as exhibited in different pre-clinical creature models of kidney disappointment. Involving a model of diabetic nephropathy in mice, the proposed system was remembered to focus on the stomach kidney hub and trigger defensive stomach microbiota, as opposed to being straightforwardly nephroprotective.

Vitis vinifera, or grape, has a place with the Vitaceae family. Grape seeds contain more than 1600 phytonutrients, including flavonoids, catechin, anthocyanins, flavonols, non-flavonoids and supportive of anthocyanidins, and their concentrates display huge organic movement. For this audit, one of the most significant of natural activities is hindrance of progress in CKD. Grape seed removal regularly acts by lightning oxidative pressure and endoplasmic reticulum stress-initiated apoptosis. Pre-clinical investigations of grape seed removals in creature models of CKD have additionally revealed superior kidney capability, diminished proteinuria and decreased podocyte cell passing. Clinical preliminaries have exhibited that grape seed extricates expanded GFR, diminished proteinuria and fatty oils, forestalled weakness, and checked plasma low-thickness lipoprotein and thrombocytopenia. There are no known unfavorable aftereffects at typical portions of grape seed extricates.

Worries of Poison levels of Plant-Based Concentrates to the Kidney

Natural products are frequently thought to be more secure than conventional medications, and a large number of our cutting edge drugs are obtained from herbs. Regardless, a few specialists are worried about their protected use. The conceivable nephrotoxicity and other ongoing or slippery wellbeing issues involving famous correlative and elective medication in various nations are not properly reported.

The most notable harmfulness or incidental effect is related with conventional Chinese home grown medication that utilizes aristolochic corrosive and incites aristolochic corrosive nephropathy (AAN). The clinical highlights of AAN are described by broad interstitial fibrosis and cylindrical decay in the kidney without clear glomerular injury. Drawn out use causes urothelial malignancies.

What's more, traditional natural cures have been ensnared in 35% of all instances in Africa. The Restorative Products Organization confined the utilization of ephedra in Australia because of its possibly poisonous impacts (stimulated heartbeat and raised pulse, heart palpitations, queasiness and retching). A few natural medications that contain explicit spices, nuts and mushrooms may likewise be related with innate nephrotoxicity. Curiously, the inborn properties of the spices are not by any means the only wellspring of spice related kidney issues.

Herb drug connections, botches in measurements and distinguishing proof, toxins inside combinations, debasement with weighty metals, and, surprisingly, conscious defilement with non-named plant removes are issues of concern. Nonetheless, with appropriate distinguishing proof, thorough pre-clinical and clinical preliminaries, severe controls on the presence of debasements inside home grown drugs, naming of measurements and contraindications, and powerful assembling strategies, the security of those consuming natural medications ought to be kept up with.

The analysts concluded: " There is no question that plants present to a great extent undiscovered sources of new CKD treatments. Clinical and preclinical preliminaries of plant removal some of the time show benefit, however some examination has likewise exhibited that plant concentrates might create constant organ brokenness when utilized for the long haul because of the presence of unsafe synthetic substances. In this way, the point of late examination is to recognize, thoroughly test pre-clinically and clinically, and keep away from such harmful results to acquire ideal restorative advantage from restorative plants. This survey might end up being a separating instrument to specialists into reciprocal and elective prescriptions to figure out the latest things of utilizing restorative plants and plant extricates for the treatment of kidney illnesses, including CKD."

CHAPTER SIX: ABOUT DIALYSIS

Dialysis is a kind of treatment that assists your body with eliminating additional liquid and side-effects from your blood when the kidneys can't. Dialysis was first utilized effectively in the 1940's and turned into a standard treatment for kidney disappointment beginning during the 1970s. From that point forward, a large number of patients have been helped by these medicines.

Dialysis should be possible in a clinic, a dialysis place, or at home. You and your primary care physician will conclude which kind of dialysis and which spot is ideal, in view of your ailment and your desires.

Dialysis is useful for two distinct circumstances:

- Acute kidney injury (AKI): an unexpected episode of kidney failure or kidney harm that occurs inside a couple of hours or days. AKI is generally treated in an emergency clinic setting with intravenous liquids (given through the vein). In serious cases, dialysis may likewise be required for a brief time frame until the kidneys improve.

- **Kidney failure:** at the point when 10-15% of your kidney capability functions well, estimated by an expected glomerular filtration rate (eGFR) of under 15 mL/min. At this stage, your kidneys are as of now not ready to keep you alive without some additional assistance. This is otherwise called end-stage kidney disease (ESKD). With kidney failure, dialysis is simply ready to do a portion crafted by healthy kidneys, however it's anything but a remedy for kidney disease. With ESRD, you will require dialysis until the end of your life or until you can get a kidney transplant.

How it functions

Dialysis plays out a portion of the obligations that your kidney for the most part does to keep your body in balance, for example,

- eliminating waste and additional liquids in your body to keep them from developing in the body
- Balancing minerals in your blood, like potassium, sodium, calcium, and bicarbonate
- assisting with managing your circulatory strain

Types

Hemodialysis (HD)

In hemodialysis, a dialyzer (separating machine) is utilized to eliminate waste and additional liquid from your blood, and afterward return the sifted blood into your body. Prior to beginning hemodialysis, a minor medical procedure is expected to make a vascular access site (opening into one of your veins), typically in your arm. This entrance site is vital to have a simple method for getting blood from your body, through the dialyzer, and back into your body. Hemodialysis should be possible at a dialysis place or at home. Medicines typically last around four hours and are completed three times each week. Certain individuals might require additional opportunity for medicines in view of their particular necessities.

Peritoneal Dialysis (PD)

In peritoneal dialysis, your blood is sifted inside your own body as opposed to utilizing a dialyzer machine. For this sort of dialysis, the covering of your mid-region or tummy region (likewise called the peritoneum) is utilized as a channel. Prior to beginning peritoneal dialysis, a minor medical procedure is expected to put a catheter (delicate cylinder) in your tummy. During every treatment, your stomach region is gradually loaded up with dialysate (a purifying liquid produced using a combination of water, salt, and different added substances) through the catheter. As your blood streams normally through the area, additional liquid and side-effects are pulled out of the veins and into the stomach region by the dialysate (practically like a magnet). Following a couple of hours, the liquid blend is depleted from your midsection utilizing the very catheter and pack that was utilized toward the start of the treatment. Peritoneal dialysis should be possible anyplace in the event that you have the provisions expected to play out the treatment.

Effectiveness

Dialysis is an exceptionally compelling treatment choice for cleaning side-effects and additional liquid off of your blood. In any case, it doesn't completely supplant every one of the kidney's capabilities, so it isn't viewed as a remedy for kidney sickness or kidney disappointment.

A wide range of dialysis are similarly successful, yet your ailment and individual inclinations might match one treatment approach better compared to other people. You and your primary care physician will examine this and conclude which kind of dialysis and which spot is ideal. You may likewise find it accommodating to converse with others who are living with dialysis to gain from their encounters.

The accompanying advances can assist with expanding the adequacy of your dialysis medicines:

- complete your therapies as per your endorsed plan
- follow your modified eating plan suggested by your kidney dietitian
- get however much active work as could be expected to support your solidarity and heart wellbeing
- talk with your dialysis supplier and drug specialist about any meds, enhancements, or natural items you are taking or are thinking about beginning
- chat with your dialysis group about any worries or aftereffects that you may have Secondary effects

Side effects

The two kinds of dialysis accompany secondary effects.
It can likewise be difficult to tell without a doubt
whether a side effect is a result of the dialysis or the kid
failure that is additionally influencing the body.

Each individual answers diversely to dialysis, and your
degree of hazard for each incidental effect will vary from
others. On the off chance that you have worries about
any of these dangers, converse with your primary care
physician and dialysis group about ways you can bring
down your gamble. Albeit these incidental effects might
sound alarming, they ought to be contrasted with the
dangers that come from proceeding to live with untreated
kidney disappointment.

Extra Contemplations

Influence on normal everyday practice

A great many people on dialysis can keep a customary daily schedule with the exception of the time required for therapies. Dialysis frequently cheers individuals up on the grounds that it assists clear the byproducts that have developed in the blood between medicines. Be that as it may, certain individuals report feeling tired after dialysis, particularly assuming that they have been seeking dialysis medicines for quite a while.

Individuals getting dialysis medicines additionally should be aware of what they eat. The particular dinner plan suggested for you might differ relying upon which kind of dialysis you get. Work with your kidney dietitian to make a feast plan that accommodates your daily schedule and way of life.

Voyaging is likewise an opportunity for individuals on dialysis. Dialysis focuses are in all aspects of the US and numerous different nations. The treatment is normalized. You should make an arrangement for dialysis medicines at another dialysis community before you go. The staff at your ongoing focus might assist you with making the arrangement. Visit the NKF Travel Tips AtoZ page for more data.

Many individuals on dialysis can return to work after they have become accustomed to dialysis. Notwithstanding, on the off chance that your occupation has a great deal of actual work (hard work, digging, and so on.), you might have to search for an alternate kind of work. Visit the NKF Working with Kidney Infection AtoZ page for more data.

It will probably take you and your family a chance to seek used to including dialysis medicines into another everyday practice.

Costs

Dialysis medicines are over the top expensive. In any case, a great many people with kidney disappointment are qualified for Federal medical care when they start dialysis. This implies the national government pays 80%

of all dialysis costs. Confidential health care coverage or state Medicaid projects may likewise assist with the expenses. Visit the NKF asset on protection choices for individuals on dialysis or with a kidney relocation to find out more.

Discomfort

You might have some inconvenience as the needles are placed into your entrance site. Over the long haul, individuals ordinarily become accustomed to being around these needles and hardware. The dialysis treatment itself is easy.

Life expectancy

It depends on your medical history and how well you follow your treatment plan, and different factors. The typical average longevity on dialysis is 5-10 years. Notwithstanding, numerous patients have lived well on dialysis for 20 or even 30 years. Converse with your medical services group about how to deal with yourself and remain sound on dialysis.

CHAPTER SEVEN: SUCCESS STORIES OF CHRONIC KIDNEY DISEASE SURVIVORS

Becca was one of the 37 million individuals living with kidney sickness, and she didn't have knowledge of it," she said. " she had been told that there was a little protein spilled in her urine but she paid little attention to it . She said assuming she knew, she would've requested further tests, particularly her kidneys. But after grabbing a hold of my lecturers about herbal, natural ways to help herself, dialysis became so easy and her kidneys are better functioning.

At the point when Patricia was unexpectedly determined to have stage 5 kidney disease, meaning her kidneys were exceptionally near disappointment or as of now had fizzled, she was quickly placed on dialysis, and burned through three years on dialysis prior to that, she had been up to date with natural remedies and herbal treatments.

"There are five phases of kidney disease. Assuming you get it sufficiently early - the vast majority, they get it at stage 3a or 3b - you can slow the movement of it, or even prevent it from advancing," she said. " If you are analyzed early, you can see a dietician, and you can track with your lab reports, and eat in like manner, and afterward by and large, carrying on with a sound way of life is the most ideal way, and staying aware of your ordinary arrangements, and getting physical."

Barry Spence was feeling the side effects of end-stage kidney illness when he was started off a transport in provincial Manitoba last month.

The 41-year old guaranteed he was crushed sitting in a peritoneal dialysis preparing room at Seven Oaks General Clinic (SOGH).

After his underlying PD catheter medical procedure was not effective, a later medical procedure worked out in a good way and Spence was nearly set to begin home dialysis.

He loaded up a transport returning to home base to Thompson where he intended to mend from his strategy and invest energy with family before his next arranged excursion to Winnipeg for dialysis preparation.

Sadly, with his kidney health quickly declining, Spence became debilitated on the transport ride home showing side effects of uremia.

"At the point when our kidneys aren't working, these poisons develop in our bodies and that adds to this large number of side effects," makes sense of SOGH nurture Elaine Schaffer who works with patients progressing onto home peritoneal dialysis. " Uremic side effects get intensified as kidney infection advances and can influence the entire body.

After Spencer found out about a few solid natural prescriptions and dietary aid, he figured out how to further develop his kidney wellbeing to a generally excellent percent. He continued to dialysis which assisted speed the accomplishment with rating. He is a constant kidney illness survivor and a cheerful family man.